T0303660

More Praise for *So Far Afield*

"What a joy to read a debut volume that is both brimming with the vigor of life and able to make a space for us to see—and mourn—the loss of it. From "each finger curl of fruit" to the place where "forever ends in a pair of arms," Speers' poems are a beautiful exploration of how we lose and find ourselves in the movements of the mind, the creation of the self and the experiences of countless varieties of love. In language at once intimate and abstract, revelatory and raunchy, these poems suggest sinews and syntax of the human heart."

> – Kirun Kapur, author of *Visiting Indira Gandhi's Palmist* (2015), winner of the 2013 Antivenom Poetry Award

"In Frederick Speers' *So Far Afield*, men drink their own hearts, fold the corners of evenings, and find themselves and each other, cleaved together and apart. An anthem to love, to the rushing feeling of being alive, and to geography both real and imagined, this collection is a record of Speers' inimitable vision of the world. From the crooked closeness of smiles about to give out, to a lonely ghost dressed in rags of hope, Speers examines a wild range of human strengths and frailties. He also creates his own language; its interruptions, contradictions and refrains mimic the meter of actual conversation and life, giving even greater depth to his lyricism. In observations at once utterly original and so true they feel familiar, Speers demonstrates the wisdom of his own line: 'again and again, we can be found.' A haunting and beautiful book."

> – Rachel DeWoskin, author of *Second Circus* (2018), *Blind* (2014), and *Big Girl Small* (2011)

"The capacity of men to love—and to love each other—intimately, with tender affection and abandon, is a constant theme in the poems of Frederick Speers' gregariously fragile and yawp-ish first collection, *So Far Afield*. As such, Walt Whitman is a presiding spirit / companion, but so, too, is James Schuyler in the poems' keenly observant, descriptive spokenness; so, too, is Gerard Manley Hopkins in the deliberate muscularity of their rhythms. These are poems meant to be read slowly aloud, every syllable savored—dancing, talking, whispering, fighting. 'May the death that lives within you die,' one notes. Palpably unguarded, old in the soul, and almost maniacally sublime, this is a book of radical open-heartedness. I love these poems for their artfulness, but also for how alive the life in them is. This isn't just a dynamite first book, it's a book of dynamite, one to return to."

—Matt Hart, author of nine books of poetry, including most recently *Radiant Action* (2016) and *Radiant Companion* (2016), co-founder and editor-in-chief of *Forklift, Ohio: A Journal of Poetry, Cooking & Light Industrial Safety*

So Far Afield

Frederick Speers

Nomadic Press
2017

Text copyright © 2017 by Frederick Speers
Cover and spot illustrations copyright © 2017 by Arthur Johnstone
Author portrait © 2017 by Arthur Johnstone

All rights reserved. No part of this book may be reproduced or transmitted in any form or
by any means, electronic or mechanical, without written permission from the publisher.

This book was made possible by a loving community of family and friends, old and new.

Requests for permission to make copies of any part of the work should be sent to
info@nomadicpress.org.

For author questions or to book a reading at your school, bookstore, or alternative
establishment, please send an email to info@nomadicpress.org.

Published by Nomadic Press, 2926 Foothill Boulevard, Oakland, California, 94601
www.nomadicpress.org

First Edition
First Printing

Printed in the United States

Library of Congress Cataloging-in-Publication Data

Speers, Frederick, 1976 –
So Far Afield / written by Frederick Speers; illustrated by Arthur Johnstone
p. cm.
Summary: *So Far Afield* is a poetic study into the queer nature of love among men—a gay
love that's been called *contra naturam*—tracing their wild desires, spiritual connections,
and unspoken encounters, from seaside to cemetery. With a voice both musical and broken,
Speers' debut collection incorporates classical lyric forms with a contemporary elliptical
style to create new narratives about our old world—a world that keeps on falling in love,
even as it's falling apart.
[1. POETRY / Subjects & Themes / Queer Studies; 2. POETRY / Subjects & Themes /
Love; 3. POETRY / American / General.] I. Title.

2017914841

ISBN: 978-0-9994471-1-6

The illustrations in this book were created using watercolor and ink on Canson paper.
The type was set in Garamond Premier Pro.
Printed and bound in the United States
Typesetting and book design by J. K. Fowler
Edited by Natasha Dennerstein and J. K. Fowler

to my husband, Chase, and my
family far and wide

CONTENTS

OVERTURE

Under the piers I stood—naked, drinking
My heart. A man
Wandering by, handsome, earthy—who drank
Nothing, drew near
Asking questions. When he left—others took
His place. I kept
Nothing from them—nor from you, my friend.

TORCH SONG

If—*if*—if I—you—leave, leave me
(Leave me) In the arms of another evening
Leave as in forever, as forever is as even
As a pair of lightly folded arms—Leave
As forever folds the evening lightly over
Forever, even as I—leaving—Who would
Leave the arms of another for me—
For insofar as forever is and is in an evening
And we, in a pair of folded arms, are—
As though forever ends in a pair of folded arms
Clutching the folded corners of the evening
Closer than evening is and no farther
From you than I—as you light out the door
On down the street, fields and over—Leave
Leave me, some other evening, lightly, even—so

NOCTURNE IN PINK AND SILVER

Distancing himself and his silence from
His silent room; and, through narrower silences of
Their split-level house, from his
Family asleep; turning the deadbolt, slowly; feeling that tenseness
Only freedom teaches; unlatching,
Then, the rusted garden gate—to where
His t-shirt, backpack, and tight Levis are seen, across
The suburban midnight,
Dashing: neither fast nor slow—only deliberate, with each step
Up through cow-paths to a low mountain pass, where grass-tufts
Give way to dirt-roads that cut through a shimmering fur
Of pine groves; to one-way gravel
And then broken-line streets, to where
Over the surging freeway he leans beside
To watch constellations learned throughout his young life
Merge into the young light from the city before him:
This pink and silver-fringed overcast
Blocking stars from their downward stares, while below,
Loves of all kind artificially glow.
Soon, on a bustling street-corner, he's sighted once more.
And the distant silences that he left he lets fade.
In their place, the self
He risked to come here for he feels he is:
Unknowing will—that is, that gemlike space in him arousing
His soul, insofar as he might be
At last aroused, and belong to a greater world than himself.
On his hairless neck this familiar and dirty wind blows:
Here he is—at last, a boy
To men, and a man to boys.
To those born knowing
You are already lost at home, know
This evening in fact happened—continues to happen
And so, lives on: In lily-scented hotel linen
Draped across a lover's lap, again and again, we can be found.

GARDEN SKETCH

Home for the first time after the first year of college:
Witness—Iceberg Roses half-submerged in sunlight nod,
Repeating themselves—row, space, row—
The day is perfect for saying he is not.
Beyond rough hedges and Rhododendron,
Neighbors trade in mulching secrets, while kids with their
Red and white kites plunge the deep-end of Heaven: all of Nature,
Taken up by other matters, as they sit; and through good,
Double-paned windows of their vinyl-sided
House, we watch them study clouds outside that separate
Together in slow abandon. From this height can we tell
He's the worst son ever for
Having told her how he felt? (Among the emptied
Clutter of closets filled with boxes, dreams diffused.) In June
Sunlight, dust rose to shadow, where it's no use
To have a future now: his old childhood room
Since filled with family pictures—framed one
After another, those unmoving smiles—while their own
Crooked kind of closeness threatens to give out.
Still, the world must wait for even that to happen—much less
For her to hold him—and not herself: it's
As though she could choose. Or forget
To. Today—on this perfect day—it will take
Thought not to say it, and lose what's now already lost.

TULIP CRAZE

First Impression
Paperwhite
Silver Heart
April Moon
Ace of Diamonds
Beelzebub
Climax
Lightning Sun
Black Twilight
Job's Memory
Orange Cloud
Green Fire
Ocean Drive
New Look

Lilac Perfections
Snowstar
Night Flight
Yellow Mask
Dark Eyes
Longfellow
White Swallow
Final Touch
Whiskey
Fringed Rhapsody
Rosy Wings
Hella Lights
Golden Spike
Peerless Pink

EDEN PARK HOTEL

Boxer-briefs, from the mirror's corner—a meaningless fling's
Arm stretched across his back; on another's arm, his hand asleep.
On the doorknob in the hall, where cleaning women sing—
Advancing—hangs DO NOT DISTURB. Once more
Sodom and Gomorrah has been revised:
Angels, more willing this time—the crowd, much less of a scene.
Rain of God's fire and brimstone: distant dreams....
A pink cheek, in bed, turns toward the elevator's chime.
To leave—and not look back—is that now the crime?
Watch the wheel spin, the story get reworked,
Followed by that endless moment when you know
Someone must get hurt.
What he must've looked like, trudging home through morning snow:
Freezing thighs, vacant mind, a figure all alone.

FOG

Everywhere. Everywhere around us, and waves
Out of nowhere between the sand and my feet. Cloaked only
By what can be seen, the sea is changing
Its tune—Love me / Love, me— / Love
Again and again it goes, without ever going away
For good: only different ways of going on and on
Forever. Different types of fog. Different kinds of shores,
Though I only ever find myself walking on this one.
The fog. The sand. The tide. As it happens.
Only thing *not* possible is the world *isn't* here.
Though the world isn't necessary. At least, not today
When all there is, is love, love, love.
If you've ever worked hard to lose your way, only to find it
Right there again, under your feet, I don't have to tell you
What I'm saying: Fog everywhere—and, the impossible waves.

NEW MOON

Disturbing force—*In solemn silence, Lord*—the issue is
And issues forth: froth, a swell, the trough and crest—
We bow our heads before thee—as one clear
Wave from my upbringing wrestles free: More to follow.
Far off, rolling purrs of Storm Petrels accompany
The quiet roar—*Maker and Father most Holy.*
Late along the shoreline, campfires extinguished.
It's not union, only a uniform dark
I wish for, no clarification—only calm:
No more calling morning, noon, and night.
(Note, the whisper on the waves this time is mine.)
For peace of mind
I will set the record straight: tonight was only
Our most recent breakup, not the most painful.
Why my call, then, and why so late? Not just to let you go—

☙

In such a night when summer swells, with songs sung low
And high, trough and crest, rough enough to feel the seaward
Pull again—but to cut off the very question of you
Before there had been words;
Before you appeared, all wondrous and what-not:
Watch, as I blow it all wide open—into one small bubble
In which this song is held, rising above the tide, now,
To rest on your bristling frown of stubble . . .
In such a night, in such a night, ten thousand summers die.
But—there will be tonight; there will be *true peace, and calm —*,
God, for now and ever—*cease.*
For, should you ever have loved me—by the morning's tide, leave no
Lasting motion for me to find, no healing
Ripple to point to, no parting to hold on to, no
"On earth as it is in heaven," no echoed *Amen*. No, don't even.

TIDAL FLATS

Confirmed by the Common Terns that plunge-dive
Exclamation marks into an August harbor; by
Luminous Moonsnails and Knobhead Whelk
By the live Periwinkle, where Ghost Crabs are flung
Among pale straws fired through marl; by each
Of the small brackish waves, recalling only
That residual chore, to carry on
And on about you; by the lonely
Laughing Gull, heading home in every direction; by
Dull Coca-Cola shards strung
Along with Brittle Stars, beneath the gauze
Of grass; by the sand-drawn
Skull I claimed to be no less than the "circumference
Of knowledge";
And by those two, clear blue eyes
That had convinced me: there are no such things as lies.

THE PINES ON FIRE ISLAND

As one sore at the base of the pine begins to pop—
I rub my arms, and yawn.
(Wave upon wave of rusting tree-tops dawn.)
In truth its loss should hardly shake this grove, packed
So much with loss: black fruiting mauves,
Globs catching needles shed in brown throngs
Aping the tarnished dieback that spires over
Shabby parapets, failing cathedrals of the cove.
Morning's haze like incense trims
Higher boughs, where lofts of redwings
Used to wake—*conk-a-ree, conk-a-ree*—though quiet
At this hour, their tune loops inside my brain, entwined
With snippets from another song—*Forget not those—Forget not*
Those who have fallen in the field—While beneath
Brightening skies—*Without shelter*—
I wait, as together the varied losses wreathe.

☙

Back to the weekend timeshare, to take my pills and sleep—
Comforter turned down; the tide recedes:
In truth one loss can't be replaced, not even by another loss
Or two that holds you a moment longer.
In my head, the scene from earlier plays on endless loop:
Squatting next to the pine, patiently I watch
As this strand of blight-drool drips from its wounded bough
And drowns a bug wandering through.
(I am not myself.)
From resistance to resistance of resistance: as one
Sore—not those—at the base of the pine—in the field—forget
Forget, forget—the needles' dead refrain!
Friends, in the meantime—perched outside
On the limb of a dream—ring
And ring: *How is it there? And you? How*
Are things—are things . . . How are—things?

TWO AND A HALF MINUTES TO MIDNIGHT

I

If the ocean isn't composed of fiery coals
I no longer know what is
I no longer know what is
And the ocean is not so composed
I no longer know what it is—I
Don't know: to turn all of it upside-down
If only for a moment, to divine natural law
(Why do the dark depths go unrecognized?)
For the ocean doesn't float in mid-air
From somewhere it fires up
The clear engine of itself—and from
Somewhere else this self-same fire
Imagines that it's there
If the ocean isn't composed of fiery coals
And moved by wild, old laws
Let's say I no longer know what to say
Though we say it anyway
With waves that flag understanding
With skeletal remains of a frigate
And an unexpected plume of gray
Extending the night clouds, unclear
Save for some tinged with reddish orange
And are those human forms, near the shore
If the ocean isn't so composed
Stay in the moment, then, a moment more
If the dark depths are no longer dark or deep
But are now closing in, clearly, from all sides
If the ocean's no longer composed of midnight
Smoldering with a deep and restless sleep
Why should we be overcome
By anything other than love
Wild love, oldest song of the known universe

The kind of knowing song that makes you
No longer know just what to say
Against the brown-red and red-orange night sky
With a smudge of clay
What isn't there to love, with clear, dark eyes
After we no longer know what to say
When all there is has already been lost
Then, and only then, from anywhere
Can we fire up the cause of our day

II

Now the only thing that makes me laugh
Is knowing I'll never laugh again
And because I'll never laugh
Again, it's fucking hilarious, I'm afraid
This being half sad, yet so positive
(Who doesn't love a lost cause?)
Go on and soak that all up
My friends, my blood
Cradled in the skull held at arm's length
Like your white mug filled with dark rum
(And tiny pink umbrella)
You sip from, now, quietly resting
Under the palm trees bent
In the shade of the evening sun
My blood, there, in bloodless terms
Flowing still with undetectable bugs
Organisms with no clear origin
Transmitting things unknowable
Like this echoed song
With no clear singer, and notes that don't form
A single chord

Yet spill across the galactic ocean, somehow
Circulating now in this skull, which you hold out
(Though suppressed by meds, these days
More whimper than bang
The dampened verse of a deathly refrain
In the tubes of my veins) And you say
What there is to say
What is there to say, my friends, tell me
Cause I'm afraid I'll never laugh again
(I mean, I'm sad to say
The fact is, I'll never laugh the way
I do when I'm with you)

III

Under the palms bent in the shade of the rising moon
Two and a half minutes to midnight
Say all of what we have to say is true
Blood-dark ocean, humid and full
Earth's crust, moving like a human skull
And then say none of it is
That it's only ever been some cosmic joke
Set in motion, well before laughter's birth
Then let's say you
Find this specter floating between the two
(Whose side are you on?)
Radiating there, between truth and the one true joke
Some lonely ghost dressed in rags of hope
Glimmering like this poor pool of moonlight
Between our closed door and the floor-boards
(It must be there, there it goes, on the other side)
Roaming the courtyard brush, among
Blank-faced statues, each sun-bleached and rain-worn

(As grief is its own reward)
Some figure hovering by the Slipper Orchids
Wearing, from time to time, a mindful overcast
That tattered gray robe
You know by heart, hanging low enough to touch—
(Whose side are you on?)
Gray mist pinked with light
When glittered stockings are peeled off
And shaken out into the flowing arroyo
As tiny reflections that float along the self
When the classic again becomes corporate
Where do we go, now
Ghost of our ghost
Under the bent palm made light by the shade of this moment

IV

I say, don't we make such a lovely pair
You not really here, and I—not altogether there
For it is this kind and phantom fact
Alone that separates me from you
Bringing us closer than we could've thought—
Although the cool rain I feel on my face
Now isn't real, and will never end
For when we pose the question of "have" or "have
Not" and the question of "you and I" or "not"
Love itself falls like a raindrop
Among the ocean already full of raindrops—
Each path leading us back
To this hidden patch of sand
While the ocean spends all night returning
Horseshoe Crabs softly upon their shields . . .
Walk with me, friend, what's done is done

Our fates are so far gone—that now
We can be vulnerable again, lying
On our backs: watch as the clouds part first
As one, then heal as two—and then, at last, depart the sky
Without our ever imagining why
And over there—there, a comet dusts the star fields

DARK HALLWAY

"Stars are falling but you still feel the same way."
– Moby, from "Landing"

In the grand scheme, of course, we are
Fools, thinking feelings hold meaning.
Look, the distances between heavenly bodies are vast:
Any affinity we have is finite;
Distances between stars are vast.
One way to appreciate this fact is by seeing
Our insignificance as singular—
Singing, all the while, that
The distance between stars and bodies is vast.
It's all we need, and not all that sad,
As nothing—nothing changes this fact.
And yet, that we can say nothing forever
To each other, over and over again, across the field, is
—The distance between our bodies is vast—
Proof that something, something does get passed,
Yes? Did you say yes?

DEER SKULL IN THE UNDERGROWTH

I spot you there, half-hidden among Birch saplings and Swamp
Rose, both of us awfully still,
Before the shadowed campsite here, in the heart of the forest,
Where the carved moon shines down with a thousand songs
I may never know. In the dark thicket all around
Lightning bugs move about: each, swallowed by the night,
Returns high above, on some branch or leaf.
I remember, as a little boy I'd catch their kind in a jar,
And watch as that poor universe blinked in and out.
Brushed with dirt, dazzled with Ragweed, your young antlers
Remain unmoved, tuning in to something well beyond us,
And your eye sockets hold nothing back.
I shift my weight on the log and adjust my sack,
A prepared thing, compact, just enough to see me through
This trip, like the luminescence each bug carries to the end.
By now, the moon has filled the air with an underlying chorus
Where did I go wrong… Where did I go wrong—
When one from the swarm floats inside the cave of your head
The way a memory can return home
To an empty apartment. Blink, and it's gone
Again: small, bright corner of the world.
Why do we love that which can't love us back?
With a stick, I move some dry, thorny vines aside
And touch your cold endurance with my fingertips.

LEAVES ON THE AIR

See how some reddish leaves have fallen only
To float again, swirling up in the vacant lot
Beneath blue clouds gathering (or departing)
And how the sunset in the river shines
Brighter with its own diminishing
For whatever's beyond the horizon seems more promising
And how could that be wrong—
Being lifted up, like a patch of fog ...
To reflect on things also amounts
To being-in-the-world
Though the senses never find common ground
Walking through a park or peering through windows:
Goodwill hand-me-downs, and thrown-together dreams abound
With scraps, love-birds ringing about their nests—
Even as we close our eyes (close them now)
Everywhere continues to fall, terrifically, into
Places, people, places—
A world of random faces one must learn by heart again
And again, though always
With different notes of longing
Like some absent-minded chorus
No one can conduct, nor keep from singing.

NORTH AMERICAN STARLING

From—no longer of—the evening air, a starling slows; descends
Past torch-red maples, Central Park—fluttering
The dusk—it folds in darker iridescences
From; no longer foreign, from sixty-four
To untold densities—to
American-made Bethlehems and Parises; from here
And there to variegated fogs, all hues
Of coal—a cloud, in fact, yet no form
Of weather—when an element of one
Flits and fits through disjointed oaks,
Alights, and turns to sing: *All the birds*
Have started nests—Except
For you and me

෨෨

As one feather shed sheds light while shadowing
The flock—which works, separately together, now
Through one gray cloud, as folks
From Rome, Indiana, flip porch-lights on … Across
Our continent of disconnected thoughts—from Richmond to
Richmond, from to Portland to Portland,
Across the heartland's Hot Springs, Springfields
—Plural as thunder, a handful
Of Hell's Gates, to where Hopes abound; across
Heart-shaped states, heavy with traffic—
Liberty, Sierra Vista, Olympia, as one broken
Scarlet of a spotlight lowers—Los Angeles—
All the birds … except—
What are we waiting for?
No longer *of* so much are we as *from*
As from this muffled, dry *wrrsh* of flight

෨෨

From municipality to multiplicity of light
Settling among the knotted branches of tonight—
No longer "a love of" and "a love of" and "a love of"
Only this one love *from*
Taking shape, seen here as from above:
Gas-lamps flickering still to fluorite strands
Wing-like, magnificent
Out through urban joints to cul-de-sacs, fresh-clipped laws, tips
Where sprawl ends—unfurling manifold
Us: And above all that, the dark we are
No longer of . . . yet
A correspondence from which arises, even now, this magic
Third note or "difference tone," a chord made so with only
The playing of any two notes: *All*
The birds have started nests—What on earth are we waiting for?

WATERFALL

Go on, say it all—all at once, from where we overflow
Part of the miraculous, where the body seeks its spirit and is so
Formed; where what is given is giving over to itself, as in
This mist spent in falling that'll never reach the earth—
From crack to wing-bones, two halves
Of a single curve narrowing into
A kind of knowing—the hand imagined
Slowly becoming this hand
Washing down my back, my head
Resting on the altar of ourselves:
Good clothes crumpled on the moon-drenched rocks.
When the spirit finds the body, it's also part
Of the miraculous, as a body can't forever call
The body home—so, go on, Love—
Look for the source outside yourself, as much as you'd like,
For then, and only then, will we draw closer—close.

GEODE

I hate—love. O, isn't it queer: Just 'cause this heart I
Feel is glistening, I break it open—and, broken, feel.

INTERLUDE BLUES

Start over, from where we were (i.e., where we *are*)
Starting over—for however long it takes
To make a heart—a fully fledged, human one
Capable of beating, breaking, being
Remade into different forms, at once incredible
And credible—enough, so it can be put down
And picked back up—Only now is it clear what time it's in
For neither its beats nor its breaks tell more
Than the tune itself—As instruments, we are
Unfinished—for you
And I, on any evening, noon, or night
Spoke of such things (such things) in any kind of mood
Any tone of voice, or no words at all—and so it is
And is—is pointless to pinpoint the heart's true form
Although, we—make a start to work from

THE LIFE OF BATHHOUSES

"...contra naturam..."
– Thomas Aquinas

Well, time's made short work of that stone wall, and—
Watch yourself on the low, Roman arches—iron gates
Hoarfrosted off their hinges;
Rusted open to the old great hall
At the end of a torch-cold hallway,
Where ivy clings to ceilings
Crowded once by gods—
Crumbled now to an overcast that sweeps over unhallowed
Grounds, and where nameless rest from more ancient worlds,
As we resume our tour:
Blow a kiss to the wall, if you'd like,
With its mortar red stained, lichened white
And pinked by mold—
Proving nothing, more or less, as it fell
Save whatever it sheltered:
It has held, having weathered itself.

༄

So let's piece whoever it was together with
However they have fallen apart:
Some fretwork here, and there—recessed lights on down the hall.
Let us approach the calling through careful mourning
(Meaning, we should be of two minds—one
To bear witness, and the other, fruit).
To find a real space
The living may inhabit with unreal loss, first
We must note: there are no documents to speak of—
And focus, instead, on the fact
Their loss is lost to us; because, however strong
Our desire is to know, the recounting of their lives
Forms only a threshold for us—

Door of shadow, door of light, through which we step—
Quiet now—to a world of men laid end-to-end
In the cold steamroom of the old Meatpacking District:

⚬ⓢ⚬

Filled, once, with divine moaning, this was the place to be,
Until an untimely death swept each life away.
Today, in what's become this room, the only
Trembling now comes from dust
Clogging the mouths of rusted pipes;
And from right outside this wall,
Faint sounds of horns rushing by ...
To unearth whoever they were
When they were together; to breathe
Deep, and believe the pain we sense was also theirs;
To locate the disembodied voices now—
"So empty ..." And, "What bars?"
A neighborhood can't help but change its tune.
Feel how temporary the things they loved were, too:
Where there used to be
Men are mounds of stone
Zoned for renewal
And strip-mall, strip-mall, strip-mall ...

⚬ⓢ⚬

What shouldn't was become? Only love
Ruins love. As long as what has been
Has been withstood, then
Those who came before us are in fact
Gods: Well-built and with
Gold rings—humble, no doubt,
Though not harmless to themselves:
Their honor endures a human wall.
Around this fountain, the path channels

Run-off, with bits of plaster, as it
Winds along the ember-hearth, coiling
Toward this moment's room—
Until a candle-flame's worth it fills up, and seeps
Through cupped hands,
Pressed to dry lips.
As long as what has been withstood surpasses what can be
Understood, how can the heart not keep overflowing stone?

ᴥ

Now here is where a thirteenth-century church once stood:
It's become a different kind of sanctuary, for
Those less saved by god than demonized
By his followers—this comely, gutted stone-husk
With some dizzying details preserved: Nothing,
Once built, can't be broken down again, then
Rebuilt—the ruins of one love
Turn up in the bones of another:
Surrounded by the faded mural of *John 13: 1–17*
It's my first time in this place: white towel
Wrapped around my waist, I stare down at my feet—
Make it the feet of some guy across the dance-floor
Decked in leather, with a humming bird tattoo
High up on his left thigh, its fluted beak
Tapping at his bedazzled codpiece—

ᴥ

(We should be of two minds—one to bear
Witness, and the other, fruit).
Crisscrossing pink lasers diffuse through the smoky air
And scribble glyphs across a cracked baptismal font
Just below a dingy frieze—when, trance-like,
A diva's voice from high-definition speakers
Possesses the floor: All

Voices run together now...
In the flash-lit dark, I listen for
Arabic. Korean. Turkish. Russian.
Spanish. Dutch. Portuguese. German.
Among whirlpools, cages, chains, and slings
Two stunning St. Andrew's Crosses flank the pulpit,
Where unrelated men air-kiss
And move about in circles, spoiling the end
Of the latest blockbuster, suffering one
Another's flashbacks, and the usual talk of evil exes.

&

As it happens, the heart keeps overflowing stone:
Pan now from *ostium* to *exitum*—
Where this handsome stranger takes my hand
And we push our way through
The crowded oratory...
Above us, frescoes with angels vault, unstripped,
While below, pumped men move in the dance-floor's pulse.
We make our way to the altar. Seen up close,
On his right shoulder, a pale bruise forms—unless,
No, another—even more fresh—tattoo;
Make it rest there, beneath the metal
Buckle of a handmade harness, half hiding
The silhouette of two lips parting—no,
I'm wrong: It's the descendant sign
In the Second House this month—Taurus,
A blue-inked bull's head, shaded just so
To make it appear as if
The skull rises above the flesh.

&

Just before dawn, another music in me stirs
Without a sound, as we continue feasting

43

On falling in love: Neon signs for spirits
Encircle the crowds, still
Dancing like beasts with glowing crowns
And bodied shields that form this moving wall—
God, what a great song—
Even a minor amplitude in
Faith can be the foundation for man's longest fall.
Beside the flaking frescoes of cherubs
And the lurking apostles who feign to look on: only
Love ruins love (we know this so well). What remains
From today can always be made
Into tomorrow: The chorus
Of one song found on the lips of another.
If this, friends, is our lineage, then
Have him take my hips, as we push further in—
Each man thinking, *Make him work for it.*

୭ଡ଼

Closing time: giant halogen lamps flicker on,
Echoing the east, through a reconstructed rose
Window framed by sleek organ pipes
Around the choir loft—as though signing
It's four o'clock / It's four o'clock
Time to step outside again, and believe a little
In the dying whirlpool of the night,
To have it swirl about us—the overflowing
Dark through which we make out pricks of fire
Too vast to take in, all at once—the entire
Bathhouse having emptied out, flooding the streets
With human builds and unearthly lust
—What shouldn't was become?—
For what's manifest can always be
Remade before our eyes, brick by brick, as we walk
One foot in front of the other—life taking us

Only so far, until we're nothing more than
Moonlight making our way home through the mist.
And even then—lord, how we kiss. And kiss.

FRUIT PLATE

As their angel unzips, and whips it out—
Eyes the shiny ten-gauge starter-hoop
(Sterilized), and then, to the female
Technician, nods;
His father—
At the kitchen counter, with fruit plate
In front of him, appearing worlds away
Or farther—
Sipping coffee
And skimming
The front page
With his right hand; while with his
Left, mechanically,
He is
Piercing, with a stainless-steel fork,
This plump, red, seedless grape.

FIELD OF POPPIES

One and Only

Heart Throb

Husbear

Papi

Slick

Creepy Guy

Good Looking

Bubble Butt

Snuggles

Boo

Lover Boy

Sweet Pea

Slam Piece

Handsome Devil

Starshine

Better Half

Love Bug

Gym Bunny

Fuck Buddy

DILF

Less Creepy Guy

Trick

Sugar Daddy

Snugs

Beau

Boy Toy

Piece of Ass

Spark of My Life

Bright Eyes

Hey You

VICTORY OF GARDENS

Man-sized compost heaps, disturbed in the distance. Listen:
It's 1 a.m. again, where we sit among constellations of men
Circulating for sex, within the reed-lined rampart called "The Fens."
Bristled skin, creamy flesh: a Chestnut near the fence
Droops, drops its seed on a moldy *STAR*, mounds
Of crumpled *HEARLD*s (one, with opened countenance, looms
Over curls of pansy on the pile's scalp). Inside loams,
Grubs thread through gourds, egg-shells, singing without a sound,
Up through glorious filth, thick and syrupy as stacks
Of flapjacks served at the all-night diner, each man
Goes for around dawn, departing one by one, while the ground
Retains some of the feeling that went on: Darkening soil,
Absorbing the rejected, with silent company and unseen toil:
Give, take; take, give—all part of the universal pattern.
Even now, over by the ringless husband
Getting his reach-around,
Up from the manure a mint sprig is sprouting.
Come, we can have courage, and have much to learn.
Let's find a spot where we won't be heard.

STILL NIGHT

At last the night stood still; and we who alter forms
Now could make certain things clear, starting with ourselves:
If I've led you to believe my thoughts were a waterfall or waves
And these strong limbs a river flowing, long ago
I learned such magic isn't real, and have since turned them back.
But my arms are open nonetheless, and will not fail you or rush.
Here, water fills water, fire burns, and blooms bloom—
While fear, love, and beauty appear to be not even of this realm;
Only that which stays as it is, is here—and us,
So long as we hold as still as the night, without saying as much.
Today, from the dark depths of this silent well
I draw new life again—and will, so long as I can,
Always with joyful sorrow, as though clinging to some key words
Keeps the deep meaning of an old song alive—
The song that drew us together, that night the night didn't move.
Song of pure intent; difficult, yet nearly true—not impossible
            to learn by heart:
Song for sheltering all who hear it from all they hear—
When, at first light, you leave once more—leaving me with fear,
            love, and beauty.
But in that time, I loved being alone with you
Having learned what it is to hold perfectly still.

TWO MEN OBSERVING THE MOON

"Here or nowhere is our heaven."
– Henry David Thoreau

If—hear me out—I'm neither here nor there;
If these phrases are merely whispered to the cold air;
If, in fact, I do all the voice-overs for my inner voice;
If my self-worth vents ultimately into an all-encompassing depth,
And that's all that's meant by individual choice
For however long we hold our collective breath;
If I point the finger at nothing in particular, and kneel
As nothing (through clouds, and the turning of the earth)
Paints a smoky, light sphere across the very field,
Which neither you nor I alone could have conceived through art
With as much perfection,
As our meeting point extends infinitely in both directions—
Then, maybe we can be, in part, convinced
Of anything—life, death, or the human condition
Our doubtful existence, our believable fictions . . .
—And, if wandering through such a night, you should find
More like-minded bodies—bring them by, so I may listen.

GREAT HORNED OWL

How do I honor you—you
Who stand beside me watching the night on either side
Move nearer with light
How do I tell you—your words—kind and not-so kind
Keep me alive
(How I wish you could see you as I've come to see you)
How do I give you
A sense of my varied and immense gratitude
How do I generalize
—How do I
Cry across this valley from the mountainside
What you must know
I feel toward you
How can I show my love for all-of-who-you-are to me
But slowly, always—and even then.

WANDERER ON A MOUNTAIN TOP

Nothing is without the sky, where whiteness forms
The sky, without a break—and the clouds
White clouds, foam-like, without a sky to see
Plainly, from every side—the emptiness, complete; nothing, there
Vast and flat as the mid-winter sea—
Nothing without the notice of white sails farther in the distance
Shifting their weightlessness from side to side
While all around the edges of this neat expanse
Light without brightness glows
So that nothing now is
Without the dull luster of opal—
All-absorbing, billowy drift of white, this
Serenity of the bleak variety
Coasting the blue-black ridge stretching north
Lighting the way to nowhere of concern
A forest or valley, who knows—
When each off-white wave draws back our gaze
Wherever we turn in this open space—
No towns in the distance are there to be found
No birds on the wind, no insects discovering mauve blooms
No sounds without you here, with me, on this trail
Where I turn my sore foot in its boot, and wait
While clods of fresh dirt roll down the mountain face—
Down into nothing more, and down into nothing great.

BALD CYPRUS

May death's needle-like leaves break off and fall away
May the death that lives within you die—and in so doing give you
        new life …
May death's breath fail to fog the glass—
In your wellspring, may death drown, and the eggs
It has laid be swallowed up by the greater death you've imagined
        for yourself
May death disappear into the dead of night
And may the dark metaphors that harbor death also fall away
Sink to the bottom of the lake, and form this talisman
        that gives new life
Unless … death must also live to keep you alive—Then
        may death
Be lost among the mirrored halls reflecting the best moments
        from your life:
When the clouded curtain falls, may there be one more encore
To enjoy, the sun, a spotlight waiting—and everyone here is
        here for you—
Then may this cure continue for others' sake, like
        love's rusty token
For after we're gone, and these words long forgotten—
A favorite rune or trusted song, in someone else's pocket.

SKULL ROCK

On the New Year's Eve of your departure, I stand watching
Snow on the cold boulder mounds, where gnarled
Arms of Joshua Trees reach
About this national park's minor attraction—Skull Rock—
Where those daring, dare—why
Not?—to climb through blank weather up. Where what falls, falls
Only as snow—a dusting, here—on broad shoulders of dirt.
Given such hope, there's no reason to be cautious now.
Adjusting for tragedies everywhere else, big and small,
Why couldn't this exact moment be flawless?
Where rope is the perfect tool. And couples with kids, heroic.
Who, after all—besides the impossible stoic,
Who himself can't imagine he's the creature imagining
There's nothing more than what is there before him—would find
This peaceable expanse of rock, tree-limb, and snowfall
Upon mountain after mountain in the distance, inadequate?
Am I, after all, incapable of leaving well enough alone?
For once in my life, can't I forget such questions?
Can I look at the rock that looks like your gaunt face
And see just the rock before me?
Is that awful to say? Awful to think? Does that make me
An awful person? And how awful
Do I have to be, before nameless gods
Come to realize they've made a grave mistake—
And that I should take your place?

GROVE

Lay down, Love, my arms: His death is to be
Let in. Cagey heart, you got me this far
Before, and now back again—through a sea
Of faces, home to this empty lot—just
Let *letting go* go, for once;
Let myself hold what one life meant—
Body of cold light, warm breath—his determined form,
Though I know it can't be held anymore
By anyone. By now
I should have learned: Love shall grieve
Within the grove of quiet ash, where it went
Once, gladly, without official say-so or belief.
As is the custom, Love, show me how
To give this giving-in the room it needs:
Nothing, nothing is set in stone, I know,
Though forever always takes its leave.
Let me see who is there but can't be seen—
For now there can be no other response.
Love, lay down. My arms. My arms.

SPIDER LILY

Near the cemetery fence a glowing bloom stands alone,
Leafless. The glowing bloom stands alone
And loneliness is the object.
The object is struggling for
A lover who doesn't show.
One lover shows only when the other
Doesn't:
Only the petals
Or these leaves,
Never both.
When the leaves flourish,
The petals have wilted;
When the flower waxes,
The leaves have fallen.
Not being together, they grow
Restless. Being restless is desire itself
And worth possessing, if only for ourselves
As we wait for the other near the cemetery fence.

WHITE RIVER

Not in the goodbye so much itself as in the greeting
Of goodbye, the real letting go, as you say (*hello*)
Rests not in the heat of the moment: When one
Decompensates—when one truly loses it—it is never
In that blind spot, where one feels full of heartache, anguish—
Not with red-eyes swollen, mouth twisted, hands wrung—
But in the months or years that follow, in
A diner, say—sitting in the middle of nowhere—where a river
Outside traces through fields, sunlight shimmering off its back—
Where a waitress smiles, and fills your water-glass—
And then, not even then—not even in a moment of kind reflection
On water filling your glass, or this river resisting the flow of itself—
But in the first bite you take of a tuna fish sandwich.

UNDER THE LEMON TREE

Decayed still-life: how to mark the moldering last
Curve of yellow-green, this white, furry orb of shadow
There, on the red brick path of our garden—
Sagging slow, like an old man's breast, back into itself—
More penicillin, at this point, than fruit.
To picture what's left for us, too, may be unhealthy;
To guess what the earth will soon rework,
A selfish pursuit: the subject,
Dark and useless. Oh so
Useless, and right there at my foot. Far-fetched,
Even, to watch the passing of such blight-touched things;
Impractical as possible. And yet clear as the sunlight
We can't see, revealing the spoiled
Figure on the ground: it becomes this perception
Of a lovely being, being undone, as each
Finger-curl of fruit, over time, relents.
To embrace death, one needs to be strong, we believe;
Strong enough, at least, as all the bitterness taken in.
And weak, too. Weak as the faint arc of light that now
On this fading rind for no real reason shines
And shines—O god, I still haven't gotten it right....
What a loss, devoting one's life to loss.
The whole subject, dark and useless,
As soon, we find it everywhere under foot—
Yet another ruin by the lemon tree.
But that young lime over there? It's doing fine:
With its fresh, if fainthearted, greenish yellow
Sheen, its shine puts them all to shame—
Without the slightest introspection
On death or (for that matter) life,
It swells imperceptibly.
Though I can't remember the last time
I didn't occupy myself with time, this time
I want you to know how I tried:

On the garden path, every evening
I practice walking toward you, as though
Through prayer: The chilled air
Filling our lungs, as the dying day
With dark clarity
Reflects on all the small things we have to say.

STAR JASMINE

Someone around this block must love the stuff.
Stumbling down garden stairwells, reeking of last night:
Light cologne of weed or skunk, yet sweeter still;
And so pungent by mid May, that, with the slightest whiff
From a stiff morning breeze
My face becomes this unbecoming twitch
Just walking down the street.
Something in me gets that I don't get it:
This dark-green dormancy springing to life, life, and more life,
When all I want is to walk to work in peace.
To learn its Latin name and Asian origins
Raises only more questions. There's so much
I don't know I don't know. And so,
Tomorrow, I promise to do things a little differently,
Breathing in the glowing commotion it makes
Outside the window—just enough, I think, until it's clear
Where it gets its power from: like those
Five-fingered blooms, with their universal invocation
To open the senses, and move beyond the self, self, self.
Someone around the block must love this stuff.

D.C. AL FINE

True, we don't need an occasion to talk
About such things;
But then, there's one before us: Scrum of gold
And red leaves, wheeling
Across the surface—and fish, probably,
Dark beneath. In fact,
Wouldn't the real loss be not to work with the scene
We've been given?
Go on, my love, my cherished one, my reason
For being—ask your questions.

ACKNOWLEDGEMENTS

Grateful acknowledgment is given to the editors of the following journals in which my poems were previously published:

AGNI (online): "Tidal Flats"
Diode Poetry Journal: "Victory Gardens" and "Eden Park Hotel"
Forklift, Ohio: A Journal of Poetry, Cooking, and Light Industrial Safety: "Interlude Blues" which appeared as "from Torch Songs"
Ofi Press Magazine: "Spider Lily"
Salamander Magazine: "White River"
The Straddler: "Leaves in the Air"; and "D.C. al Fine," which appeared as "Leaves on the Pond"
Syzygy: "Two Men Observing the Moon" and "North American Starling"

My deep appreciation to the Vermont Studio Center for its support and community over the years, as well as to my loving friends, who mean the world to me and my poetry—MK Chavez, Jamie Cash, Mikola De Roo, Natasha Dennerstein, Rachel DeWoskin, Zayd Dohrn, Valerie Duff, Marvin Dunson III, Carolina Ebeid, Aaron Fogel, J. K. Fowler, Njambi Good, Matt Hart, Kirun Kapur, Joseph Ligammari, Susan Mizruchi, Jeff Pethybridge, Carl Phillips, Robert Pinsky, Mara Servitas, Jacob Strautmann, Jonathan Tze, Frank Verlizzo, Mūkoma wa Ngũgĩ, and Rosanna Warren.

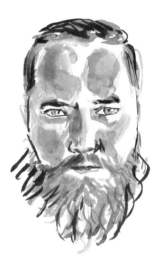

FREDERICK SPEERS grew up in the Blue Ridge mountains of Virginia, and he has since lived in Washington D.C., Boston, Amsterdam, New York City, the Bay Area, and Denver, where he lives now with his husband and their Jack Russell Terrier. Fred is the founding editor of *Jam Tarts Literary Magazine*, and the first recipient of the Fitzpatrick / Thoreau Fellowship from the Vermont Studio Center. A graduate of Boston University's Creative Writing Program, Fred has since worked as an editor for nearly two decades, for both high-tech companies and publishers, including Oxford University Press, where he published, among other books, the second edition of Oxford's *Anthology of Modern and Contemporary American Poetry*. Fred's own poetry has appeared in a handful of journals, and *So Far Afield* is his first collection.